Published By Robert Corbin

@ Hazel Bonny

Acid Watcher Diet Cookbook: Tasty & Nutritious

Recipes to Acid Reflux With Natural Remedies

All Right RESERVED

ISBN 978-1-7385954-1-9

TABLE OF CONTENTS

Quick Pepper Quiche 1

Sweet Chicken Salad 3

Smoothie With Bananas And Ginger For Energy 6

Fruit And Pine Nut With Couscous 7

Heartburn-Friendly Tomato Sauce-Free Lasagna 9

Heartburn-Friendly Baked Chicken Parmesan 13

Green Smoothie 15

Apple Lemonade 16

Melon Smoothie 17

Strawberry Banana Flax Smoothie 18

Almond Cookies 20

Chocolate, Almond, Nut And Coconut Cookies 22

Banana Nut Pancakes 24

Blueberry Or Strawberry Pancakes 26

Black Bean And Cilantro Soup 29

Flavorful Cantaloupe Gazpacho 30

Quench-The-Fire Quiche With Tofu And Mushrooms ... 31

Easy Baked Chicken 35

Butternut Squash Soup 37

Instant Polenta With Sesame Seed 40

Banana Oatmeal Pancakes 42

Chicken Stir Fry Easy Dinner Recipe 45

Sesame Encrusted Baked Chicken Tenders 48

Spiky Green-Smoothie 50

Green Energizer 51

Maple Ginger Overnight Oats 52

Banana Almond Flax Smoothie 54

Stuffed Chickpea Flour Pancakes 56

Buckwheat Pancakes With Nettle Sauce 59

Egg-And-Cheese-Stuffed Tomatoes 61

Shirred Eggs With Crumbled Cheddar Topping 64

Creamy Hummus 66

Watermelon And Ginger Granite 67

Oatmeal Marc's Way 69

Muesli-Style Oatmeal 70

Simple Chicken Matzo Ball Soup 72

Spinach Artichoke Soup 74

Crunchy-Wheat French Toast 76

Raisin Bran Muffins 78

Fall Veggie Pizza 80

Tomato-Free Pasta Sauce 85

Green Wheat Smoothie. 89

Bok Choy Smoothie 90

Green Aloe Vera Smoothie 92

Cantaloupe Ginger Chia Puddings 93

Savory Pie With Red Lentils 95

Savory Pie With Potatoes And Creamy Mushrooms 100

Mini Quiches 103

Sesame Lettuce Wraps 105

Chicken Noodle Soup Ingredients: 107

Rice Noodle Medley 109

Instant Polenta With Sesame Seeds 110

Sautéed Shrimp With Angel Hair Pasta 112

Cream Of Mushroom Soup 115

Stewed Chicken And Dumplings 118

Carrot Salad 122

Spinach And Arugula With Apples And Pears 124

Vegetarian Sweet Potato And Lentil Salad 126

Split Pea Soup 128

Cucumber Salad 130

Peachy Smoothie 132

Smear Smoothie 133

Easy Overnight Oats With Cinnamon 134

Pear, Ginger And Almond Yogurt Parfait 136

Energy Cookies With Oats And Raisins 137

Soft Fruit Plumcake 140

Chicken Breast With Scallions, Snap Peas, And Beans . 142

Spiced Stuffed Peppers 144

Flank Steak With Chimichurri 147

Low Fodmap Coleslaw 149

Oatmeal-Crusted Rosemary Salmon 151

Quick Pepper Quiche

Ingredients:

- ¼ tsp smoked paprika
- 2 cage-free eggs
- 1 small onion
- 1 clove garlic
- ½ red bell pepper
- 1 tbsp extra virgin olive oil

Directions:

1. Finely chop onion, garlic and red bell pepper.
2. Pour extra virgin olive oil into a pan over medium heat.
3. Crack eggs and pour into a small bowl. Combine with onion, garlic and red bell pepper and whisk until mixed together.

4. Pour contents of bowl into pan and add smoked paprika.
5. Scramble until desired doneness. Serve.

Sweet Chicken Salad

Ingredients:

Date syrup

- 1 cup pitted dates
- 1 cup water

Salad

- 1 red bell pepper
- 1 yellow bell pepper
- ½ cup walnuts
- 1 cup strawberries
- 1 cup kiwi
- 4 pieces grass-fed chicken thighs, coarsely chopped
- 1 tbsp extra virgin olive oil

- 7 oz bag Romaine lettuce

Directions:

1. For Date Syrup, split the dates down the middle, remove the pits, and place in a bowl with 1 cup water. Place this mixture in the fridge overnight. Stir occasionally if you are able to.
2. Preheat oven to 375. Take the chopped chicken thighs and coat them in olive oil. Place them on a baking dish, cover with aluminum foil, and place them in the oven for 30 minutes.
3. Chop the peppers and slice the strawberries and kiwi.
4. When the chicken has cooked for 30 minutes, remove the aluminum foil and cook for another 15 minutes. After 15 minutes, drizzle half the date syrup mixture over the chicken and cook another 5 minutes.

5. Place the romaine lettuce, peppers, walnuts, strawberries and kiwis in a bowl and toss.
6. Remove chicken from oven and place into the bowl.
7. Drizzle the remaining date syrup over the finished dish and toss.
8. Serve immediately or chill 20 minutes and serve.

Smoothie With Bananas And Ginger For Energy

Ingredients:

- 1 quart of yogurt
- 1/2 teaspoon fresh ginger, peeled and finely grated
- 2 tbsp. honey or brown sugar (optional)
- 1/2 cup of ice
- 2 quarts of milk
- 3 ripe bananas

Directions:
1. Blend the ice, milk, yogurt, bananas, and ginger in a blender.
2. Blend until completely smooth.
3. Add in sugar as desired.

Fruit And Pine Nut With Couscous

Ingredients:

- 1 quart of orange juice
- 1/4 teaspoon ginger (grated or micro planed)
- 2 tbsp. raw sugar or Honey
- Two tablespoons raisins
- 1/4 teaspoon allspice
- 1 cup Tabouli or alternative couscous (packed)
- A single banana (diced in tiny pieces)
- A single apple (smoothened with a grater)
- Salt
- One tablespoon roasted pine nuts

Directions:

1. Preheat a skillet over medium-high heat.
2. Toss in the couscous and toast for a few minutes. Or until the scent is released and the color turns golden brown.
3. Place in a medium bowl.
4. Simmer the orange juice and pour it over the couscous.
5. Wrap the bowl with plastic wrap and set it aside for 5 minutes.
6. Use a fork to separate the grains in the couscous.
7. Add the banana, apple, and raisins to the couscous when cold or at room temperature.
8. Add Honey or sugar, ginger, raisins, spices, salt, and stir everything together.
9. Transfer to a plate. Put in 1 tsp roasted pine nuts, if desired.

Heartburn-Friendly Tomato Sauce-Free Lasagna

Ingredients:

- 1 tablespoon all-purpose flour
- 2 tablespoons butter
- 1/2 cup high-quality Parmesan cheese, shredded
- Salt and freshly ground pepper, to taste
- 1 1/2 cups skim mozzarella cheese, grated
- 12 ounces wide lasagna noodles
- Nonstick cooking spray
- 12 ounces very lean ground beef (ground round or ground sirloin)
- 1/2 cup low-sodium beef broth
- 1/4 cup low-fat cream cheese

- 1 1/4 cups skim milk or 1% milk, divided

Directions:

1. Heat oven to 375F.
2. Bring a large pot of salted water to a boil. Add the lasagna noodles and cook according to package instructions, or just until tender. Drain well. While the noodles are cooking, continue with the rest of the recipe.
3. Spray cooking spray onto a large, non-stick pan. Add the ground beef and cook over medium heat until it is browned and no longer pink. Drain the liquid.
4. In a large bowl, add the browned beef and beef broth. Mix together.
5. To make the low-fat Alfredo sauce, combine cream cheese, about one-fourth of the milk, and flour in a small mixing bowl. Beat until well-blended. Slowly pour in the remaining milk and beat until smooth.

6. Melt butter in a large, nonstick saucepan over medium heat.
7. Add the milk-cream cheese mixture.
8. Cook for about 4 minutes, stirring constantly until the sauce has thickened.
9. Stir in the Parmesan cheese. Add salt and pepper, to taste. Turn off the heat.
10. Spread 1 cup of the low-fat Alfredo sauce over the bottom of a 13x9-inch baking pan.
11. Add three strips of cooked lasagna noodles to cover the sauce. Spread half the beef mixture on top.
12. Lay down another three strips of lasagna noodles. Spread the remaining beef mixture on top. Then, lay down the remaining three strips of lasagna noodles.
13. Spread the very top with the remaining Alfredo sauce. Sprinkle with mozzarella cheese.

14. Bake for 25 to 35 minutes until bubbly and golden. Remove from heat and let cool for 3-4 minutes before serving.

Heartburn-Friendly Baked Chicken Parmesan

Ingredients:

- Dash of salt
- 4 boneless, skinless chicken breasts
- 4 teaspoons olive oil
- 1/2 cup seasoned breadcrumbs
- 3 tablespoons Parmesan cheese, grated
- Dash of Italian seasoning

Directions:
1. Heat oven to 375 F.
2. Lightly coat a baking dish with vegetable cooking spray.
3. In a small bowl, add the Parmesan cheese, seasoned breadcrumbs, Italian seasoning, and salt. Mix well.

4. Pat chicken breasts dry, lay on a plate, and coat them with olive oil.
5. Dredge chicken breasts on both sides in the breadcrumb mixture, and transfer to the baking dish.
6. Sprinkle any remaining breadcrumb mixture over the chicken.
7. Bake uncovered for 35 to 45 minutes, or until done.

Green Smoothie

Ingredients:

- ½ cup of water
- ½ cup of collard greens
- ½ cup of spinach
- ½ bell pepper (green)
- 1 kale leaves

Directions:

1. Thoroughly wash all fruits and veggies.
2. Using a blender, start by blending the vegetables. Combine the fruit in a blender.
3. Transfer the contents of the bowl to a serving glass and enjoy.

Apple Lemonade

Ingredients:

- ½ cucumber (quartered)
- ½ carrot
- ½ apple (quartered)
- ½ lemon

Directions:
1. Thoroughly wash all of the fruits and vegetables
2. Using a blender, start by blending the vegetables.
3. Combine the fruit in a blender.
4. Transfer the contents of the bowl to a serving glass and enjoy.

Melon Smoothie

Ingredients:

- 1 lime, juiced
- 2 tbsp sugar
- ¼ cantaloupe - peeled, seeded and cubed
- ¼ honeydew melon - peeled, seeded and cubed

Directions:

1. Mix cantaloupe, honeydew, lime juice, and sugar in a blender.
2. Blend until completely smooth. Fill glasses with the mixture and serve.

Strawberry Banana Flax Smoothie

Ingredients:

- 1 cup of spinach
- Serve With
- 4 slice bread, whole wheat
- 1/4 cup of peanut butter, all-natural
- 1 cup of Greek yogurt, plain
- 2 medium banana
- 1 cup of strawberries, frozen, unsweetened
- 1/4 cup of flaxseed, ground

Directions:

1. In a high-powered blender, add all smoothie INGREDIENTS:. (If your blender won't mix it,

add a little water at a time until it does, but try as thick as possible to keep it thick.)
2. After toasting the bread, slather it with peanut butter.
3. Serve right away.

Almond Cookies

Ingredients:

- 100 g of powdered sugar
- 50 g of flour
- 2 egg whites
- 20 g of water
- 400 g of peeled almonds
- 400 g of light brown sugar
- 1 teaspoon of yeast

Directions:
1. Finely chop the almonds with 350 g of brown sugar.
2. In a saucepan, over low heat, dissolve 50 g of sugar in 20 g of water.

3. When the syrup is ready, add it to the almond mixture and the yeast, flour, and 50 g of powdered sugar.
4. The mixture obtained must rest at room temperature for at least 12 hours covered with a damp cloth.
5. After 12 hours, whisk the egg whites with 50 g of powdered sugar and mix them with the almond mixture (they are gradually incorporated by mixing them from the bottom up).
6. Work until it is soft and homogeneous.
7. Obtain some loaves that you will cut into small pieces and to which you will give the shape of the almond.
8. Bake in the oven at 110 ° for about ten minutes. Let cool before serving with a sprinkling of icing sugar.
9. Store them in a tin box to keep them longer.

Chocolate, Almond, Nut And Coconut Cookies

Ingredients:

- 50 g of walnut kernels
- 30 g of shredded coconut
- 50 g of whole coconut sugar
- 1 egg white whipped until stiff
- the peel of 1 organic orange
- 100 g of dark chocolate
- 50 g of shelled almonds
- 1 pinch of salt

Directions:
1. Put the diced chocolate and the other dry INGREDIENTS:, including the orange peel, in the mixer.

2. Blend everything for a few minutes until it is reduced to a powder.
3. You will get a rather lumpy mixture. Meanwhile, whip the egg white until stiff and add it to the dough, mixing carefully.
4. Using a spoon, form balls of the mixture and place them on a baking tray lined with parchment paper.
5. Try to distance them from each other because they will widen during cooking.
6. Bake the cookies at 150 ° for 25 minutes. Let them cool before removing them.

Banana Nut Pancakes

Ingredients:

- 1 medium banana, mashed

- 1 tablespoon baking powder

- 1 cup rice flour (or substitute corn, chickpea, or custard flour) Nonstick cooking shower, as needed

- 1/2 cup milk

- 2 huge eggs

- 11/2 tablespoons margarine, softened

- 1 cup coarsely cleaved walnuts

Directions:
1. In the bowl of a food processor, join milk, eggs, spread, and banana.

2. Gradually add baking powder and flour until fused. Don't overmix.
3. Prepare a medium dish or frying pan with nonstick splash.
4. Heat dish on medium. Pour in hitter 1/2-cup at a time.
5. Sprinkle nuts on top of each cake.
6. Turn when flapjacks start to rise on top. Put on a warm platter.
7. Present with newly whipped cream, extra cut bananas, or the product of your choice.

Blueberry Or Strawberry Pancakes

Ingredients:

- 1/2 cup milk
- 2 enormous eggs
- 1 1/2 tablespoons margarine, dissolved
- 1 tablespoon baking powder
- 1 cup rice flour (or substitute corn, chickpea, or custard flour) Nonstick cooking splash, as needed
- 4 1/2 16 ounces blueberries or strawberries
- 1 tablespoon granulated sugar
- 1 teaspoon ground orange zest
- Freezing Fruit in Its Prime

Directions:

1. There's nothing like blueberry pie in Ja nuary, and not the fruit that comes loaded with sugar syrup in a can.
2. When fresh blueberries are available, just rinse a quart and dry on paper towels.
3. Place the berries on a cookie sheet in the freezer for 30 minutes and then put them in a plastic bag for future use.
4. In a huge bowl, blend natural product, sugar, and orange zing.
5. Crush with a potato masher or mortar and pestle.
6. In the bowl of a food processor, consolidate milk, eggs, and spread.
7. Gradually add baking powder and flour until fused. Don't overmix.
8. Prepare a medium dish or frying pan with nonstick splash.

9. Heat dish on medium. Pour flapjack hitter by 1/2-cup segments into the dish and spoon a few berries on top.
10. Turn when air pockets ascend to the highest point of the cakes, and brown the opposite side.
11. You will get a few caramelization from the sugar and organic product it's delightful.
12. Top with more berries and whipped cream to serve, if desired.

Black Bean And Cilantro Soup

Ingredients:

- ½ cup fresh cilantro
- Salt to taste
- 1 tbsp. nonfat sour cream
- 8 oz. canned black beans
- 1 pint chicken stock

Directions:
1. Bring the chicken stock to a boil. Add the beans, cilantro, and salt.
2. Cook 30 minutes on low heat.
3. Blend with a hand blender to the desired consistency.
4. Season, as needed.
5. Serve in a soup bowl and garnish with 1 tsp. nonfat sour cream and a sprig of cilantro.

Flavorful Cantaloupe Gazpacho

Ingredients:

- 2 tbsp. brown sugar or agave sugar
- 2 tbsp. port wine
- Dusting of fine-grated nutmeg
- 1 lb. (2 cups) cantaloupe (skin removed, seeded, cut into 1-inch pieces)

Directions:
1. Mix the cantaloupe, sugar, and port. Place in the freezer for about 4 hours.
2. Blend in a blender.
3. Finish with a dusting of nutmeg.
4. Serve immediately in a shot glass or small cup.

Quench-The-Fire Quiche With Tofu And Mushrooms

Ingredients:

- 1 egg yolk
- Salt to taste
- 1 3¼4 cups all-purpose flour
- 5 Tbsp water
- 2 Tbsp butter
- 2 egg yolks
- Salt to taste
- 2 Tbsp Parmesan cheese
- 1 cup (6 oz) silken tofu, soft
- ½ cup of the water from the tofu

- 1 Tbsp butter

- ¼ tsp grated nutmeg

- 2 Tbsp chopped parsley or cilantro

- 1 ½ cups (4 oz) shitake mushrooms (stems removed, washed, and cut into thin strips)

- ½ cup dry porcini mushrooms (re-hydrated in cold water for an hour, drained)

- 1 ½ cups (4 oz) domestic mushrooms (remove ¼ inch from the stem and slice thin)

Directions:
1. Place the tofu and water in a blender and process until smooth.
2. Add the two egg yolks and the Parmesan cheese.
3. Season with salt to taste.
4. In a glass or plastic measuring cup, combine the water, butter, and salt.

5. Melt the butter and let it cool.
6. In a bowl, add the flour, one egg yolk, and the mixture of water, salt, and butter.
7. Use a plastic scraper to cut the butter into the flour.
8. When the mixture is completely combined, form into a circle about 1 inch thick and 6 inches in diameter.
9. Wrap in plastic wrap and refrigerate for 30 minutes.
10. Spray the inside of an 8-inch tart mold with non-stick spray, or rub with butter. Roll out the dough on a well-floured flat surface until the diameter is about 2 inches larger than the tart mold all the way around and the same thickness throughout.
11. Place the dough in the mold and refrigerate for 20 minutes or until dough is leathery.
12. Place parchment paper or aluminum foil on the cold tart shell and fill tart with dried beans

or special metal balls used for "blind baking" (pre-baking).
13. Cook in the oven at 350°F for 10–15 minutes or until the dough becomes chalky.
14. Remove the beans or special balls as well as the parchment paper or aluminum foil.
15. Return to the oven until the dough is golden brown.
16. Allow to cool.
17. Sauté the mushrooms in butter and a little bit of salt until all the moisture from them is released and they turn golden brown.
18. Add the sautéed mushrooms to the bottom of the cooked tart.
19. Cover with the tofu custard.
20. Sprinkle with chopped parsley or cilantro and nutmeg.
21. Return to the oven until custard sets and top is golden brown, approximately 30 minutes.
22. Serve immediately.

Easy Baked Chicken

Ingredients:

- 4 stems rosemary
- 3 tbsp extra-virgin olive oil
- 1 lemon
- ½ cup organic chicken stock
- 4 pieces grass-fed chicken thighs
- 4 cloves garlic

Directions:
1. Preheat oven to 450 degrees.
2. Strip the leaves from the rosemary and crush the garlic.
3. Grate the lemon into zest and juice and separate the two.

4. Place chicken on a baking dish. Add garlic, rosemary, lemon zest, and olive oil.
5. Toss chicken to coat thoroughly and roast (uncovered) 20 minutes.
6. After 20 minutes of roasting, add chicken broth and lemon juice. Turn over chicken.
7. Return to oven, turn oven off and let sit 5 minutes longer.
8. Remove from oven and place on serving dish, pouring pan juices over the chicken.
9. Serve immediately or chill 20 minutes and serve.

Butternut Squash Soup

Ingredients:

- 1 cinnamon stick

- Celtic sea salt, to taste

- 2 tablespoons shelled pumpkin seeds (toasted or raw)

- 2 tablespoons ghee (or coconut oil or bacon fat)

- 2 tablespoons coconut oil (or bacon fat)

- 1 medium-large butternut squash (about 2 cups diced)

- 2 cups chicken stock (or veggie stock)

- 1/2 cup coconut milk (optional)

- 1/2 onion (white, yellow or sweet)

- 1/2 large carrot

- 1/2 celery stalk

- 1/2 teaspoon ground coriander (optional)

Directions:

1. Heat oven to 375 degrees F. Heat medium cast iron pan over medium-high heat. Add fat to hot oiled pan.
2. Peel squash and remove seeds. Dice and add to hot oiled pan with salt, to taste.
3. Sauté until golden, about 3 - 4 minutes. Place pan in oven and roast until browned on all sides, about 15 minutes.
4. Heat medium pot over medium-low heat. Add coconut oil to hot pot.
5. Peel and dice onion, celery and carrot.
6. Add to hot oiled pot with cinnamon stick, salt and pepper to taste.
7. Sauté until soft but not browned, about 10 minutes.

8. Remove squash from oven and let cool slightly.
9. Add food processor or high-speed blender and process until puréed.
10. Add chicken broth and coriander (optional) to pot. Increase heat to medium and bring to boil. Simmer about 5 minutes.
11. Stir in squash purée and simmer about 10 minutes. Discard cinnamon stick.
12. Add mixture to food processor or high-speed blender and purée until smooth.
13. Or blend with immerse or stick blender until smooth.
14. Transfer mixture back to hot pot and stir in coconut milk (optional). Transfer to serving dish.
15. Sprinkle with pumpkin seeds and cracked black pepper. Serve hot.

Instant Polenta With Sesame Seed

Ingredients:

- 1 tbsp. orange juice

- 1/2 teaspoon vanilla extract

- season with salt to taste

- 1 tbsp. sesame seeds (golden brown after toasting in a pan)

- ¾ of a cup of instant polenta or cornmeal

- 3 cups of whole milk (or lower-fat milk if you prefer)

- 3 tbsp. sugar (brown)

Directions:
1. Bring the milk to a boil in a saucepan.
2. To avoid lumps, add the polenta or cornmeal and stir quickly.

3. Cook until the sauce has thickened to a creamy consistency.
4. Just before serving, add the sugar, salt, vanilla, and orange essence.
5. Toss with sesame seeds and serve in a dish.

Banana Oatmeal Pancakes

Ingredients:

- 1/2 cup flour made from oats
- 1/2 cup flour (all-purpose)
- 1 tbsp. baking soda
- 1/2 teaspoon salt
- 1/8 teaspoon nutmeg
- 3 big eggs
- 4 ripe bananas
- 2 tbsp. brown sugar (mild)
- 3 tablespoons (1 ounce) non-fat sour cream or buttermilk
- 2 tablespoon of butter maple syrup

Directions:
1. Combine the light brown sugar, oat flour, all-purpose flour, baking powder, salt, and nutmeg in a mixing bowl.
2. Combine the sour cream or buttermilk, eggs, and bananas in a mixing bowl.
3. If you feel the mixture is too thick, add a few tablespoons of milk at a time until you get the desired consistency.
4. Heat a nonstick skillet over low to medium heat. Rub a little butter in a paper towel and wipe the surface.
5. If there's any excess butter, brush with the paper towel
6. Use the same paper towel to re-butter before cooking the second time.
7. Pour a tiny amount of batter into the pan with a spoon.

8. When the underside of the pancake is golden brown, flip it and cook until no more bubbles or wetness appear.
9. Keep the pancakes heated until they're all done.
10. Drizzle with maple syrup and garnish with chopped apples.

Chicken Stir Fry Easy Dinner Recipe

Ingredients:

- 4 0 z. green onion cut into 1 in length
- 4 oz. snow peas
- 1 red bell pepper sliced
- 1 teaspoon grated fresh ginger
- 6 skinless boneless chicken thighs cut into bite size pieces
- 8 - 10 oz. rice noodles or thin spagetthi
- 3 tablespoon + 1 teaspoon olive oil
- 1/2 cup store bought or homemade chicken broth
- 1/4 cup soy sauce
- 1 tablespoon sherry cooking wine or rice wine

- 1 teaspoon corn starch

- splash of sesame oil

Directions:

1. Bring a large pot of salted water to a boil. Add the noodles and cook according to Directions: on the package.
2. Drain and stir in 1 teaspoon of olive oil. Set aside.
3. In a small mixing bowl combine chicken broth, soy sauce, sherry wine and corn starch. Mix and set aside.
4. In a large skillet over medium/high heat, heat 1 tablespoon of olive oil.
5. Add green onion, sliced red bell pepper, snow peas and grated ginger.
6. Stir-fry until tender, about 3-5 minutes. Transfer to a plate.
7. Add 2 tablespoons of olive oil to the skillet and heat on the medium/high heat.

8. Divide chicken in two batches, stir-fry each batch of chicken until chicken is cooked thru about 5 minutes.
9. Add vegetables, noodles and broth mixture and stir-fry for 2 minutes or until noodles are heated thru.
10. Serve warm with a splash of sesame seed oil and soy sauce for seasoning. Serve warm and enjoy!

Sesame Encrusted Baked Chicken Tenders

Ingredients:

- 2 tsp sesame oil
- 2 tsp low sodium soy sauce
- 6 tbsp toasted sesame seeds
- 1/2 tsp kosher salt
- 1/4 cup panko
- 8 chicken tenderloins, 18 oz total
- 3/4 tsp kosher salt and black pepper, to taste
- olive oil spray

Directions:

1. Preheat oven to 425°F. Spray a baking sheet with non-stick oil spray.

2. Combine the sesame oil and soy sauce in a bowl, and the sesame seeds, salt and panko in another.
3. Place chicken in the bowl with the oil and soy sauce, then into the sesame seed mixture to coat well.
4. Place on the baking sheet; lightly spray the top of the chicken with oil spray and bake 8 to 10 minutes, until slightly browned on the bottom.
5. Turn over and cook another 4 - 5 minutes or until cooked through and the edges are crisp.
6. Serve over rice with more soy sauce, if desired.

Spiky Green-Smoothie

Ingredients:

- 2 peeled banana
- 2 stalks celery
- 1 quartered cucumber
- 1 cup of spinach
- 1 small-sized carrot

Directions:

1. Thoroughly wash all the fruits and vegetables in cold water.
2. Using a blender, start by blending the vegetables. Combine the fruit in a blender.
3. Transfer the contents of the bowl to a serving glass and enjoy.

Green Energizer

Ingredients:

- ½ quartered cucumber
- ¼ cup grapes
- ½ cored apple (green)
- ¼ inch slice of ginger

Directions:
1. Thoroughly wash all the fruits.
2. Put the fruit in a blender and process it.
3. Transfer the contents of the bowl to a serving glass and savor.

Maple Ginger Overnight Oats

Ingredients:

- 1 tsp ground cinnamon
- 2¼ non-dairy milk
- 10.6 oz Vanilla Forager Project Cashewgurt
- ¼ cup of raisins
- 1 carrot
- 1 oz fresh ginger
- 2 cups of gluten-free rolled oats
- 2 tbsp agave

Directions:
1. Make the oats the night before
2. Carrots should be peeled and grated. Ginger should be peeled and minced.

3. Mix the oats, grated carrot, chopped ginger, agave, cinnamon, non-dairy milk, and a sprinkle of salt in a big mixing bowl or container with a cover.
4. Cover and chill the oats for at least 8 hours or overnight.
5. Overnight oats should be divided among four serving plates. Cashewgurt and raisins go on top of the maple ginger overnight oats.

Banana Almond Flax Smoothie

Ingredients:

- 4 Tbsp ground flaxseed meal
- 4 tsp honey
- 12 - 16 drops almond extract*
- 16 ice cubes (optional)
- 4 medium well ripened banana, peeled diced into pieces, frozen
- 2.6 cup of unsweetened almond milk
- 1.33 cup of fat free plain Greek yogurt
- 6 Tbsp creamy almond butter

Directions:

1. Add banana, almond milk, Greek yogurt, almond butter, ground flaxseed, honey, and

almond extract to a blender and mix until smooth.
2. If desired, add ice to the blender and mix until smooth. Serve right away.

Stuffed Chickpea Flour Pancakes

Ingredients:

- 3 heaping tablespoons of chickpea flour
- 2 tablespoons of oil and 1 pinch of salt
- 1 pinch of nutmeg
- 300 ml of partially skimmed milk
- 3 heaping tablespoons of spelled flour
- 2 heaping tablespoons of corn starch

For the stuffing

- ½ small leek
- 2 teaspoons of flour
- 2 teaspoons of lemon juice
- 4 tablespoons of oil and 1 pinch of salt

- 1 small thistle (about 200 g) already cleaned

- 1 slice of clean pumpkin

Directions:

1. For the batter: dissolve the flour and starch in a little milk, then gradually pour the remaining liquid and oil, beating with a whisk.
2. When the cream is thick and fluid, add the salt and nutmeg. Let it sit for 20-30 minutes.
3. For the filling: blanch the thistle in 500 ml of water where you have diluted the lemon and flour.
4. Wash the leek and slice it thinly. Sauté it in a pan with 1 tablespoon of oil and 3 of water for 4-5 minutes, then add the coarsely grated pumpkin and the shredded thistle.
5. After another 4-5 minutes turn off the heat.
6. Mix the batter. Just grease a non-stick pan and pour a ladle of the mixture into a thin layer.

7. Cook the crepes for a few minutes on both sides.
8. Stuff them and close them in a bundle. Serve hot.

Buckwheat Pancakes With Nettle Sauce

Ingredients:

- 400 ml of soy milk
- 3 tablespoons of white flour
- oil
- 250 g of buckwheat flour
- 150 g of nettle tops
- salt

Directions:
1. Put the flour in a bowl with the water needed to have a semi-fluid batter.
2. Add salt, stir and let it rest for 30 minutes. Wash the nettles and blanch them for 5 minutes in a little salted water.
3. Remove them with a slotted spoon and set them aside.

4. Measure out 100 ml of their liquid (save the rest for other preparations).
5. First, toast the white flour in a saucepan; first, pour the hot nettle water and then, always stirring and, little by little, the previously heated milk.
6. Let the sauce thicken over low heat, then add the coarsely chopped nettles.
7. Season with salt and season with a tablespoon and a half of oil.
8. Heat a little oil in a pan and cook a ladle of batter at a time until you have not too thin crepes. Serve with the nettle sauce.

Egg-And-Cheese-Stuffed Tomatoes

Ingredients:

- 1 teaspoon ground dark pepper
- 1 1/2 teaspoons ground paprika
- 1 teaspoon dried oregano
- 1 teaspoon ground cumin
- 8 enormous eggs
- 1/2 cup ground Monterey jack or cheddar
- 8 medium tomatoes
- 1/4 cup butter
- 2 cloves garlic, minced
- 1 teaspoon salt

- 8 teaspoons sans gluten chile cake crumbs Priceless Heirlooms

Directions:

1. There are good tomatoes in the supermarket and good tomatoes in cans, but the best tomatoes are homegrown.
2. Recently there has been a trend toward growing ancient varieties of tomato.
3. These "heirlooms," as they are called, have more flavor—having sweetness paired with acid—than ordinary tomatoes do. You can buy the seeds and grow them yourself, and some green markets have them too.
4. Cut off the highest points of the tomatoes, center, and utilize a melon hotshot to scoop out seeds and mash.
5. Put tomatoes on a baking sheet covered with material paper or showered with nonstick spray.
6. Preheat stove to 350°F.

7. In a little container, heat margarine on medium and sauté garlic until fragrant.
8. While it's cooking, combine as one salt, dark pepper, paprika, oregano, and cumin in a little bowl.
9. Rub the inner parts of the tomatoes with 1/2 the flavor combination.
10. Spoon the margarine and garlic combination inside the tomatoes.
11. Sprinkle with residual zest combination, saving a piece for preparing the eggs.
12. Break an egg into every tomato. Sprinkle with held flavor blend.
13. Freely spoon cheddar over the eggs, then, at that point, sprinkle 1 teaspoon chile cake scraps over each tomato.
14. Bake for 20 minutes. The tomatoes should in any case be firm, the eggs delicate, the cheddar softened, and the bread scraps browned.

Shirred Eggs With Crumbled Cheddar Topping

Ingredients:

- 12 enormous eggs

- Salt and ground dark pepper, to taste

- 1/4 cup butter

- 3/4 cup ground Cheddar cheese

- Nonstick cooking shower, depending on the situation an additional

- An Elegant Touch

Directions:
1. If you are having a crowd of people to brunch, place ramekins on a baking sheet and bake for 10 minutes.
2. Then, serve with a big bowl of fruit on the side.

3. You can use glass custard cups, but individual ramekins made of white porcelain are more elegant.
4. Preheat stove to 350°F. Get ready 12 little (4-ounce) ramekins or 6 bigger (6-ounce) ones with nonstick splash. Put the ramekins on a baking sheet.
5. Break 1 egg into every one of 12 or 2 eggs into every one of 6 huge ramekins.
6. Sprinkle the eggs with salt and pepper and dab with spread.
7. Sprinkle with Cheddar cheese.
8. Bake for 8-12 minutes, or to wanted doneness. Serve immediately.

Creamy Hummus

Ingredients:

- 2 tbsp. olive oil
- ¼ tsp. sesame oil
- ½ tsp. salt
- 1 can (19 oz.) canned chickpeas (drained and washed twice)
- 1 cup chicken stock

Directions:

1. Place the chickpeas in a food processor and add the chicken stock, olive oil, sesame oil, and salt.
2. Process until smooth.
3. Add chicken stock as needed.
4. Serve cold with toast points, oven-toasted corn chips, or small wedges of flatbread.

Watermelon And Ginger Granite

Ingredients:

- 1 pinch ground nutmeg
- 1 tsp. fresh ginger
- 1 tsp. salt
- ½ tsp. lemon zest
- 3 cups seedless watermelon juice (blended)
- 1 cup water
- ½ cup honey
- 1 whole clove

Directions:

1. Bring the water, honey, clove, nutmeg, ginger, salt, and lemon zest to a boil. Allow to cool, then strain.

2. Add the syrup to the watermelon juice.
3. Place the juice in a bowl that can be put in the freezer, and freeze 3 hours.
4. Stir every 15 minutes with a sauce whisk.

Oatmeal Marc's Way

Ingredients:

- ½ tsp vanilla extract
- Pinch of nutmeg (remember, it's strong!)
- 4 Tbsp light brown sugar, packed
- 1 cup oatmeal (3 oz, rolled or instant, toasted)
- 1 cup milk
- ⅓ tsp salt

Directions:
1. Bring the milk to a boil in a saucepan.
2. Add the salt, oatmeal, vanilla extract, nutmeg, and sugar.
3. Return to a simmer while stirring.
4. Cook 5 minutes. (Cooking time depends on type and brand of oatmeal.)

Muesli-Style Oatmeal

Ingredients:

- ½ banana, diced or sliced
- ½ golden apple, peeled and diced
- Pinch of salt
- 2 tsp sugar or honey
- 1 cup instant oatmeal
- 1 cup milk
- 2 Tbsp raisins (covered with water, brought to a boil and drained)

Directions:
1. The evening before (or at least two hours before), mix the oatmeal, milk, raisins, salt, and sugar (or honey) together in a bowl.
2. Cover and place in the refrigerator.

3. Add the fruit just before serving.
4. If the mix is too thick, add milk as needed.

Simple Chicken Matzo Ball Soup

Ingredients:

- 1 cup almond flour
- 2 cage-free egg yolks
- 3/4 teaspoon Celtic sea salt
- 16 oz (1 lb) chicken pieces
- 2 cups chicken stock (or vegetable stock)

Directions:

1. In a medium mixing bowl, beat eggs and salt until light and frothy, about 2 minutes.
2. Sift almond flour into bowl and mix until dough comes together.
3. Cover dough with parchment, if preferred, and refrigerate 2 - 4 hours.

4. Heat medium pot over medium heat. Add 1 teaspoon salt to large pot of water and bring to boil.
5. Place chicken in hot pot skin-side down. Brown chicken on all sides, about 15 minutes.
6. Remove dough from refrigerator and roll into balls.
7. Carefully place dough balls in boiling water. Reduce heat to low, cover and simmer 20 minutes, until cooked through.
8. Add chicken too browned chicken stock. Cook about 15 minutes.
9. Remove chicken and chop, then add back to pot.
10. Transfer matzo balls to serving dish with slotted spoon.
11. Ladle heated chicken stock over matzo balls and serve hot.

Spinach Artichoke Soup

Ingredients:

- 1/2 small onion (yellow or white)

- 1 garlic clove

- 2 teaspoons Celtic sea salt

- 1 tablespoon ghee (or bacon fat or coconut oil)

- 2 cups vegetable broth (or chicken broth)

- 1 can (13.5 oz) full-fat coconut milk

- 4 cups spinach leaves

- 1 1/2 cups artichoke hearts (canned or jarred, drained)

Directions:

1. Heat medium pot over medium heat. Add fat to hot pot.
2. Peel and thinly slice onion. Peel and finely grate or mince garlic. Add to hot oiled pot and sauté until tender and translucent, about 5 minutes.
3. Fill pot with spinach and stir to wilt. Continue until all spinach is added. Stir in salt.
4. Chop artichoke hearts and add to pot with veggie broth and coconut milk. Stir to combine.
5. Bring to simmer and heat through, about 8 - 10 minutes.
6. Transfer to serving dish and serve hot.

Crunchy-Wheat French Toast

Ingredients:

- 1/2 cup of milk
- 1/2 cup of flavored yogurt
- A quarter teaspoon of vanilla extract
- 2 tbsp. sugar (brown)
- 2 tablespoon of butter (or pan spray)
- 7 white bread slices
- 1/2 cup of total mashed cereal
- 3 big eggs
- Salt
- To taste, honey or maple syrup

Directions:

1. Whisk together the eggs, vanilla extract, brown sugar, yogurt, and milk in a mixing dish.
2. Place two pieces of bread in the bowl, making sure they don't overlap each other.
3. Flip the slices over when they become soaked with the mixture in procedure 1.
4. Heat a nonstick skillet over medium heat. Using a paper towel that has been dampened with butter, wipe the bottom of the pan.
5. Sprinkle a third of the cereal into the pan, then top with the bread.
6. Cook until golden brown on both sides. Follow the Directions: for the leftover bread.
7. Serve with honey or maple syrup as desired.

Raisin Bran Muffins

Ingredients:

- A single egg
- 1/3 cup of yogurt
- 1 tbsp. Flax seed (milled)
- 3 tbsp. Sugar (brown)
- A third of a cup of bran cereal
- 1/2 cup flour (all-purpose)
- 1 and 1/2 tablespoons baking powder
- 2 tbsp. Dark raisins (or other dried non-citrus fruit)
- A quarter-cup of whole milk (you can use lower-fat milk if you desire)
- Season with salt to taste

- Half golden delicious or gala apple

Directions:
1. Bring the milk to a boil in a small saucepan and pour over the raisins.
2. Combine the flaxseed, sugar, cereal, flour, baking powder, and salt in a mixing dish.
3. Whisk together the egg, apple, milk mixture, and yogurt in a separate container.
4. Using a whisk, combine the egg mixture and the dry INGREDIENTS:.
5. Spoon the batter into muffin tins that have been greased or coated with cooking spray.
6. Sprayed with nonstick cooking spray or covered with paper cups,
7. cook for at least 15 to 20 minutes at 350°F, or until golden brown.
8. Set aside for a few minutes to cool.

Fall Veggie Pizza

Ingredients:

Toppings:

- 4-5 shiitake mushrooms thinly sliced

- 1 1/2 cups shredded mozzarella

- 3 tablespoons heavy cream

- Freshly ground pepper

- Crushed red pepper for garnish

- Olive oil

- 1/4 squash

- seeds and skin removed, cut into cubes

- Kosher salt

- 1/2 bunch kale thinly sliced

Pizza dough:

- 1 teaspoon brown sugar
- 1 teaspoon Yeast
- 1/2 cup + 1 tablespoon warm water
- 1 1/2 cups all-purpose flour
- 1 teaspoon kosher salt
- 1 teaspoon olive oil for brushing crust

Directions:
1. Preheat your oven to 450 - 475 degrees F.
2. Place a pizza stone or baking steel in the oven.

To make the veggies:
3. In a medium skillet, set over medium heat, add the olive oil. When warm, add the cubed squash. Sprinkle with a bit of salt and allow to cook for about 5 to 7 minutes until tender with a fork. Transfer to a bowl and set aside.

4. Add a teaspoon of olive oil more to the skillet. Add the kale and red pepper and season with a few pinches of salt; cook for about 2 to 3 minutes, until the kale is wilted and bright green. Transfer to a bowl and set aside. Repeat with the shiitake mushrooms, cooking them for about 5 minutes in more olive oil, if needed. And then set aside.

To make the pizza dough:

1. In the bowl of a stand-up mixer with the dough hook (you could also do this in a large bowl and knead the dough by hand), add the flour, salt, brown sugar and Yeast. Mix the dry ingredients together until everything is thoroughly combined. Next, pour in the water and turn the machine to medium speed. The dough will go from shaggy to a cohesive ball. Knead on medium speed for 2 minutes, until the dough is smooth. If you're doing this by

hand, you'll need to knead the dough for about 5 minutes.

2. Remove from the dough and form into a ball. Dust the counter with a bit of flour; place the dough atop the flour and dust its top with flour, too. Allow dough to rise for 10 minutes.

To assemble the pizza:

3. Roll out the pizza dough until it's in an even layer (about a 10-inch round, using the bottom of a clean baking sheet works too). Dust the bottom of the baking sheet liberally with cornmeal or corn flour. Place the pizza dough atop the bottom of the baking sheet and then assemble.

4. Spread out the heavy cream into a very thin layer. Top with an even layer of cheese, a few rounds of freshly ground pepper and a few pinches of salt. Spread out the squash, kale, peppers and mushrooms. Brush the edges of the pizza crust with olive oil.

5. Using the baking sheet like a pizza peel, swiftly slide the pizza off the baking sheet and onto the baking steel/pizza stone. Bake for 10 to 12 minutes and until the edges of the pizza crust are lightly golden brown. Remove from the oven and sprinkle the top with crushed red pepper. Slice up and serve.

Tomato-Free Pasta Sauce

Ingredients:

- 2 cups of bone or vegetable broth (or more as needed)

- 7–10 fresh basil leaves

- 3–4 tbsp of grapeseed oil or extra virgin olive oil

- 1 tsp each of garlic powder and onion powder (omit if unable to tolerate)

- 1/2 teaspoon of dried oregano

- 1 tsp of salt to add to sauce, plus a little more to season vegetables while cooking

- 3 medium celery stalks

- 3 medium carrots, peeled

- 2 medium zucchinis

- 1 medium beet

- 1/2 a small-medium turnip, peeled

- Pepper to taste

Directions:

1. Preheat oven to 400 degrees F.
2. Peel the carrots and turnip. Cut the leafy tops close to the top of the beet, and trim the ends off of the zucchini, celery, carrots and turnip. Cut vegetables (except beet) into two-inch chunks. you can either cook all of the turnip or set the raw half that won't be used aside for later use. There's no need peeling the beet, as the skin is very tough to peel when raw. Peel it once it is cooked and slightly cooled.
3. Spread the cut up zucchini, carrots, celery, turnip and out onto a large rimmed baking

sheet lined with parchment paper. Drizzle with 2-3 tbsps of grapeseed or olive oil and sprinkle with desired amount of salt and pepper, then cover using parchment paper, tucking it snugly underneath.
4. Wash the beet using a vegetable brush, then pat dry.
5. Place in a baking dish lined with parchment paper and drizzle with 1 tbsp of olive oil.
6. Cover using parchment paper, tucking the ends underneath.
7. Place vegetables in preheated oven and cook until they are tender and can be easily pierced with a fork.
8. Stir the carrots, zucchini, celery, and turnip occasionally while cooking.
9. Once the beet is done cooking, let it cool slightly. Once cool, submerge it in a bowl of cold water and peel off the outer layer.

10. Cut it in half and place that half in a high-speed blender or food processor.
11. Feel free to add more if you want a deeper red color (keep in mind this will add a more earthy flavor to the sauce). Save the leftover beet for salads or other meals.
12. Add the remaining cooked vegetables, broth, and fresh basil to the blender.
13. Process until you have a smooth consistency.
14. Add the blended liquid to a saucepan along with the oregano, garlic powder, onion powder, salt, and pepper.
15. Cook on medium-low for 4-5 minutes while stirring. Add more broth as needed for a thinner consistency.
16. Remove from heat and serve with pasta or use as tomato/marinara sauce replacement.

Green Wheat Smoothie.

Ingredients:

- ½ small bunch of wheatgrass
- 1 peeled kiwi
- ½ sliced cucumber
- 2 medium strawberries

Directions:
1. Thoroughly wash all the fruits and veggies.
2. Using a blender, start by blending the vegetables.
3. Combine the fruit in a blender.
4. Transfer the contents of the bowl to a serving glass and enjoy.

Bok Choy Smoothie

Ingredients:

- ½ cup filtered water

- ½ tbsp. ground raw flax seeds

- ½ cup coconut water

- ½ mango

- 1 shredded head of Bok Choy

- ½ tbsp. olive oil.

- ½ papaya

- ½ tsp. kale powder

Directions:
1. Thoroughly wash all the fruits and veggies.
2. Using a blender, start by blending the vegetables.

3. Combine the fruit in a blender.
4. Transfer the contents of the bowl to a serving glass and enjoy.

Green Aloe Vera Smoothie

Ingredients:

- 150 g baby spinach leaves
- 300–450g cucumber (not peeled)
- 3 ripe and creamy banana
- juice of 3 kaffir lime (or 1 1/2 lime)
- 450ml of water
- 210 g fresh aloe vera (just the gel)
- 3/4 avocado
- 300 g green frozen grapes

Directions:
1. In a beater, mix together all INGREDIENTS: & mix until smooth.
2. Enjoy!

Cantaloupe Ginger Chia Puddings

Ingredients:

- 2 to 3 stevia packets as need or omit for Whole30
- 3/4 tsp ground ginger
- ¼ tsp ground turmeric
- 1/2 cup of chia seeds
- 1 tbsp shredded unsweetened coconut
- 12 oz ripe soft cantaloupe cubed (about 2.5 cups of – reserve .5 cup of to dice)
- 1 cup of unsweetened almond milk
- ¼ cup of unflavored collagen powder may omit without substitution needed

Directions:

1. Blend 2 cups of diced cantaloupe with almond milk in a blender until smooth.
2. Collagen powder, stevia (if you want it sweeter), ginger, and turmeric are all good additions.
3. Blend until completely smooth.
4. Add chia seeds to the mix. Pulse the blender lightly to mix the INGREDIENTS:.
5. Fill three 12-ounce (minimum) jars or containers with the mixture. Refrigerate for 15 minutes to gel.
6. Remove the remaining cantaloupe and cocoon shreds out from the oven and top.
7. Enjoy! Meal prepped and refrigerated for up to four days.

Savory Pie With Red Lentils

Ingredients:

For the base

- 3 tablespoons of extra virgin olive oil
- A teaspoon of natural yeast
- A teaspoon of whole sea salt
- 250 g wholemeal flour
- Water q.s.

For the filling

- Half a small pepper
- 2 sage leaves
- Extra virgin olive oil as needed
- Whole sea salt to taste

- Water or vegetable broth to taste

- 3 medium potatoes

- 2 glasses of red lentils

- A clove of garlic

- A slice of ginger

To garnish the surface of the cake

- Sesame seeds

- Poppy seeds

- chopped almonds to taste

Directions:
1. In a large bowl, pour the flour, salt, and yeast and mix well.
2. Make a hole in the center in which to put the oil and, a little at a time, the water needed to knead.

3. Work vigorously until you have obtained a compact but soft, elastic, and not stiff dough.
4. Let it rest for 30 minutes in the fridge. In a saucepan, boil some water with a handful of coarse salt and the unpeeled potatoes.
5. Cook them until they are soft. Drain them, let them cool and peel them. With a puree or a fork, mash them well.
6. Mix well and set aside. In the meantime, put a drizzle of oil in a saucepan, heat and fry the whole clove of crushed garlic and the chili pepper, add a little water, then add the finely chopped ginger, the sage, and the lentils previously washed under running water.
7. Mix well and add the hot water or vegetable broth necessary to cover the lentils. Salt.
8. Set aside more hot water or broth, which will be added during cooking. Usually, in 15-20 minutes, they are cooked, do not worry if they

fall apart slightly. The flavor given to the cake does not vary. After cooking, let them cool.
9. Roll out your base with the help of a rolling pin until you get an elastic dough, not too thin because it must support and give body to the cake.
10. Line a baking sheet with parchment paper and lay the base on top, cutting off the excess edge, which you can use to prepare decorative strips for the surface.
11. After removing the garlic and sage leaves, add the lentils to the potatoes. Mix well, seasoning with salt.
12. Place the filling on the base, pour over a cascade of sesame seeds, chopped almonds, and poppy seeds.
13. If you want, lay the puff pastry strips on top of the cake, forming the characteristic grid.
14. Add a drizzle of oil on the surface and bake at 200 ° for about 40 minutes.

15. Let it cool down a bit before serving.
16. This savory pie is excellent when accompanied by raw and cooked seasonal vegetables.

Savory Pie With Potatoes And Creamy Mushrooms

Ingredients:

- 6 medium potatoes
- 200 g of mushrooms
- 100 g of sour cream
- 150 g of ricotta
- 2 cloves of garlic
- 1 teaspoon of marjoram
- 2 teaspoons of sweet paprika
- 250 g of wholemeal flour
- 3 tablespoons of sourdough
- Soya milk

- 1 teaspoon of brown sugar

- 2 tablespoons of oil

- Sea salt

Directions:
1. Mix the flour with the sourdough, a little salt, and the lukewarm milk necessary to have a firm and homogeneous dough.
2. Knead it for a long time on a table, wrap it into a ball and let it rise in a warm place for 4-5 hours.
3. Meanwhile, wash the potatoes and steam them with the peel.
4. While these are getting warm, peel the mushrooms and stew them in a pan with minced garlic, paprika, marjoram, and a little salt.
5. When soft, add the cream and crumbled goat cheese.

6. Peel the potatoes and cut them into slices about 1 cm thick.
7. Roll out two thirds of the dough and use it to line a floured, rectangular, or round, high mold.
8. Spread the potatoes inside, cover with mushrooms.
9. Roll out the rest of the dough so that it covers the entire surface.
10. Seal the edges well, brush with a little warm milk and bake at 180 degrees for 30-35 minutes. Serve the cake hot.

Mini Quiches

Ingredients:

- 1/2 cup ground Jarlsb erg cheese
- 1/4 cup minced prosciutto or smoked ham
- 2/3 cup weighty cream
- 1/8 teaspoon ground nutmeg
- Nonstick cooking shower, as needed
- 1 (16-ounce) bundle sans gluten pie outside blend 2 huge eggs
- 2 tablespoons minced new chives Freshly ground dark pepper, to taste

Directions:

1. Preheat broiler to 325°F. Splash a 12-cup small scale biscuit dish with nonstick spray.

2. Prepare the pie outside layer blend as per box bearings.
3. Carry out daintily. With the floured edge of a juice glass or a 2" roll shaper, cut batter into 12 adjusts and line the biscuit cups with dough.
4. Pulse the excess fixings in a food processor until combined.
5. Fill the cups 3/4 full with the cheddar mixture.
6. Bake for around 10 minutes, or until set. Let rest for 5 minutes.
7. Cautiously lift the quiches from the cups. Serve warm.

Sesame Lettuce Wraps

Ingredients:

- 2 tablespoons ground gingerroot

- 1 pound ground chicken

- 1/2 cup sans gluten soy sauce

- 1 (5-ounce) can water chestnuts, hacked

- 1 teaspoon squashed red pepper flakes

- 1/2 cup cleaved new cilantro 1 tablespoon sesame seeds

- 1 tablespoon vegetable oil 2 cloves garlic, minced

- 2 green onions, chopped

- 1 huge head Boston or spread lettuce, leaves separated

Directions:
1. Heat oil in a huge container; add garlic, green onion, and ginger and sauté around 3 minutes.
2. Add ground chicken to the dish and extra oil if necessary.
3. Then, at that point, add soy sauce, water chestnuts, and red pepper drops.
4. Cook until chicken is brown and disintegrating separated, around 5 minutes.
5. When chicken is cooked, add slashed cilantro and sesame seeds right away.
6. Serve chicken combination in a serving bowl with lettuce leaves as an afterthought for scooping.

Chicken Noodle Soup Ingredients:

Ingredients:

- 4 low-sodium chicken bouillon cubes
- 1/2 teaspoon thyme
- 1/2 teaspoon salt
- 3 ounces uncooked egg noodles
- 2 cups diced, cooked boneless skinless chicken breasts
- 2 cups frozen peas
- 1/2 tablespoon olive oil
- 1 cup trimmed and chopped celery
- 2 quarts water
- 2 cups peeled and chopped carrots

Directions:

1. Add 1/2 tablespoon olive oil to a large pot.
2. Add 2 cup trimmed and chopped celery and sauté over a medium-high heat until translucent.
3. Add 2 quarts water, 2 cups peeled and chopped carrots, 4 low-fat chicken bouillon cubes, 1/2 teaspoon thyme, and 1/2 teaspoon salt. Bring to a boil.
4. Add 2 cups (3 ounces) large egg noodles to the boiling water. Stir.
5. Return to a boil, reduce heat and cook for 8 minutes or until noodles are tender.
6. Add 2 cups diced, cooked boneless skinless chicken breast meat and 2 cups frozen peas.
7. Return to a boil, reduce heat, cover and simmer over medium-low heat for 5 to 10 minutes.

Rice Noodle Medley

Ingredients:

- 1 1/2 cup medium noodles
- 3 cup chicken or vegetable broth
- Salt and pepper to taste
- 1 cup rice uncooked
- 1 tbsp butter

Directions:

1. In large nonstick pot coated with nonstick cooking spray, brown rice in butter, stirring.
2. Add noodles, broth, salt, and pepper.
3. Bring mixture to boil, reduce heat, and cook, covered, for 20-30 minutes, or until rice and noodles are done.

Instant Polenta With Sesame Seeds

Ingredients:

- 3 cups whole milk (or lower-fat milk if you prefer)//
- 3 Tbsp brown sugar
- 1 tsp orange extract
- ½ tsp vanilla extract
- Salt to taste
- ¾ cup instant polenta or corn meal
- 1 Tbsp sesame seeds (toast slowly in a pan until golden brown)

Directions:
1. Bring the milk to a boil.
2. Add the polenta or corn meal and whisk vigorously to prevent lumps.

3. Cook until you get a creamy consistency.
4. Add the sugar, salt, and vanilla and orange extract just before serving.
5. Serve in a bowl and sprinkle with sesame seeds.

Sautéed Shrimp With Angel Hair Pasta

Ingredients:

- 1 cup chicken stock

- 1 (8 oz) bottle clam juice

- 5 sprigs thyme (washed, stems removed, chopped fine)

- ½ cup parsley (washed, stems removed, chopped fine)

- 2 tsp sesame seeds (toasted to an amber color)

- 1 lb shrimp (16 to 20 shrimps per lb, shelled and de-veined)

- ¾ lb angel hair pasta (capellini)

- 1 lb snow peas (tips removed, cut into 1-inch diamond shape by cutting on the bias)

- 1 cup carrots (peeled and grated or cut on a mandolin to make long thin sticks)
- 2 Tbsp extra virgin olive oil

Directions:
1. Fill a large pot with water and bring to a boil. Add salt.
2. Add the pasta and cook for about 3–4 minutes. Drain.
3. Heat a non-stick pan with 1 Tbsp of the olive oil.
4. Sear the shrimp until the flesh is opaque on both sides, approximately 4–6 minutes. Remove the shrimp and keep warm.
5. Drain the excess oil and add the second tablespoon of oil to the pan. Sear the snow peas and carrots for about 1 minute.
6. Add clam juice, chicken stock, thyme, parsley, and half of the sesame seeds, and bring to a simmer.

7. Add the pasta and shrimp, and toss. Add salt as needed.
8. Serve in a soup bowl or deep dish, and sprinkle with the remaining sesame seeds.
9. Garnish with a few shrimp and a sprig of thyme.

Cream Of Mushroom Soup

Ingredients:

- 1/2 onion (yellow or white)
- 1 garlic clove
- 2 teaspoons Celtic sea salt
- 2 tablespoons ghee (or bacon fat or coconut oil)
- 3 cups vegetable broth (or chicken broth)
- 1 can (13.5 oz) full-fat coconut milk
- 4 cups mushrooms (white, baby bella, etc.)

Directions:

1. Heat large pot over medium-high heat. Add 1 tablespoon fat to hot pot.
2. Slice 1 cup mushrooms and add to pot.

3. Sauté until lightly browned and tender, about 5 minutes.
4. Remove from pot and set aside.
5. Add remaining fat to hot pot. Reduce heat to medium.
6. Peel and chop onions and garlic. Add to hot oiled pot and sauté until fragrant and lightly browned, about 5 minutes.
7. Add whole mushrooms to pot and sauté until lightly browned and tender, about 8 - 10 minutes.
8. Transfer mushrooms, onion and garlic to food processor or high-speed blender with vegetable broth, coconut milk and salt. Process until smooth, about 1 - 2 minutes.
9. Or add vegetable broth, coconut milk, salt and pepper to pot and purée with immersion blender.
10. Heat pot over medium heat. Add reserved sliced mushrooms to pot and stir to combine.

11. Bring to simmer and heat through, about 8 - 10 minutes.
12. Transfer to serving dish and serve hot.

Stewed Chicken And Dumplings

Ingredients:

- 4 bay leaves
- 1 1/2 tablespoons dried thyme (or 4 sprigs fresh thyme)
- 1/2 teaspoon dried oregano
- 1 teaspoon paprika
- 1 tablespoon Celtic sea salt
- 2 lb whole chicken (innards removed)
- 6 - 10 cups water
- 3 carrots
- 3 celery stalks
- 1 small white onion (or yellow onion)

Dumplings

- 1/2 teaspoon baking soda
- 1/4 teaspoon ground bay leaf
- 1 teaspoon dried thyme
- 1/2 teaspoon ground white pepper (or ground black pepper)
- 1 teaspoon Celtic sea salt
- Nut milk (or chicken broth or stock)
- 3 cups almond flour
- 1/2 cup arrowroot powder
- 2 cage-free egg
- 1/2 cup coconut oil, chilled (or coconut or cacao butter, room temperature)

Directions:

1. Heat large pot over medium-high heat. Place chicken breast-down in hot pot. Sear chicken and turn to brown and render out fat for about 15 minutes.
2. Chop carrots and celery. Peel onion and mince. Add to chicken with salt and spices. Sauté about 2 minutes.
3. Add enough water to pot to cover chicken. Increase heat to high and bring to a boil. Reduce heat to medium and simmer about 30 minutes. Place lid loosely over pot to prevent splatter, if necessary.
4. For Dumplings, sift almond flour and arrowroot into medium mixing bowl. Cut in solid oil or butter with fork until crumbly mixture forms. Add egg, salt and spices, baking soda, and enough nut milk or chicken broth from pot to bring together soft, slightly sticky dough.

5. Carefully remove chicken from pot with long utensil and set aside. Use utensils to remove skin from chicken. Carve chicken into desired pieces and place back in back.
6. Use spoon or scoop to gently drop dough into pot. Cover with well fitting lid and let simmer about 15 - 20 minutes, until Dumplings and chicken are cooked through. Gently stir soup to periodically prevent Dumplings from sticking. Turn over any Dumplings that are not submerged.
7. Remove from heat and transfer to serving dish. Serve hot.

Carrot Salad

Ingredients:

- 1 tsp dried oregano

- 2 Tbsp. brown sugar

- 2 tsp. Olive oil

- ¼ tsp. salt

- 1 lb. carrots (peeled, trimmed, and grated)

- ¼ lb. mesclun greens

- 2 Tbsp. raisins

- 2 Tbsp. orange juice

Directions:
1. Mix the raisins, orange juice, oregano, brown sugar, olive oil, and salt in a bowl.
2. Let it sit for about 5 minutes.

3. Pour the dressing over the carrots and mix thoroughly.
4. Season with additional salt, if needed.
5. Dish with a few mescluns leaves as desired.

Spinach And Arugula With Apples And Pears

Ingredients:

- 3 Tbsp. orange juice

- One golden delicious or red apple (peeled and cut into half-inch cubes)

- 1 Tbsp. grated Parmesan cheese

- 1 tsp toasted sesame seeds, toasted

- Salt to taste

- 2 cups of spinach

- 1 cup of arugula

Directions:
1. Pour the orange juice over the apples and pears to keep them from turning brown.
2. Wash the spinach and arugula several times until clean using a salad spinner or put the

greens into a large bowl filled with cold water, remove and repeat as needed.
3. Wash very well until all the sands at the bottom have been removed.
4. Dry very well; a salad spinner will help you do this faster.
5. Toast the sesame seeds in a pan on the stovetop or in the oven until golden brown.
6. Move them to a big bowl immediately to prevent them from burning.
7. Mix the spinach, arugula, apple, pear, Parmesan cheese, orange juice, and salt.
8. Dish and serve with sesame seed.

Vegetarian Sweet Potato And Lentil Salad

Ingredients:

- 2 Tbsp. Of Roquefort cheese

- ½ tsp. cardamom

- 8 oz. (2 cups) asparagus (peel the bottom 3 inches of the stem, cut into 1-inch pieces)

- ¼ cup fresh parsley (washed, stems removed, chopped coarsely)

- 1 Tbsp. fresh thyme (wash, remove the stems, diced)

- 2 Tbsp. fresh oregano (wash, remove the stems removed, diced)

- 1½ lb. (5 cups) sweet potato (peeled and cut into ½-inch pieces)

- 1 Tbsp. olive oil

- ½ cup of lentils

- 3 cups of vegetable stock

Directions:
1. Cook the lentils in 3 cups of vegetable stock for 45 minutes or until soft.
2. Cook asparagus in boiling salted water until smooth.
3. Place in ice-cold water to cool down and drain
4. Fry the sweet potatoes with the olive oil in a nonstick frying pan
5. Filter the lentils, and mix in a bowl with the Roquefort cheese and ground cardamom.
6. Put in the lentils, parsley, thyme, oregano, and asparagus to the potatoes.
7. Serve

Split Pea Soup

Ingredients:

- 2 to 3 diced carrots
- 1 TBSP dried chopped onion
- 1 bay leaf
- 1/2 Tsp. thyme
- 1/2 Tsp. ginger
- 1/2 Tsp. pepper
- 1/2 Tsp. marjoram
- 1 ham bone
- 1-pound split peas
- 8 cups low sodium chicken broth
- 1 cup chopped celery

- 1/4 Tsp. dried mustard

Directions:
1. Rinse peas thoroughly and inspect and pick off all debris.
2. In a large stockpot, bring chicken broth to a boil.
3. Add ham bone and simmer for 45 minutes.
4. Remove ham bone and allow to cool.
5. Add cleaned peas, all seasonings, and remaining ingredients to the pan, and return to a boil.
6. Reduce heat to a low simmer and cover the pan.
7. Simmer on low for at least 1hour or until the peas almost disintegrate.
8. Stir often to avoid burning, and if the soup gets too thick, add more broth.
9. When ready to serve, pick the meat off the ham bone and return to the pot, stir well, and ladle into soup bowls.

Cucumber Salad

Ingredients:

- 1/4 cup fresh or dried dill weed
- 4 large firm cucumbers, thinly sliced
- 1 stalk celery, thinly sliced
- 1 carrot, scraped and thinly sliced
- 2 cups white vinegar
- 1 cup of water
- 1/2 cup sugar (or adjusted amount of sugar substitute)
- 1 Tsp. Kosher Salt

Directions:

1. Bring vinegar, water, sugar, and dill to a boil a day before serving.

2. Meanwhile, layer the vegetables in a medium-sized bowl.
3. Pour the boiling vinegar mixture over the vegetables.
4. Cover, cool, and then refrigerate overnight.
5. Serve cold in small fruit dishes.

Peachy Smoothie

Ingredients:

- 1 tsp. maguey syrup
- 1 banana, shredded
- 1 cup coconut water
- 3 spinach leaves
- 1 soft ripe peach

Directions:
1. Thoroughly wash all the fruits and veggies.
2. Using a blender, start by blending the vegetables.
3. Combine the fruit in a blender.
4. Transfer the contents of the bowl to a serving glass and enjoy.

Smear Smoothie

Ingredients:

- ½ bunch of kale
- ½ cup water
- ½ ripe pear (shredded after being cored)
- ½ cup apple juice

Directions:
1. Thoroughly wash all the fruits and veggies.
2. Using a blender, start by blending the vegetables.
3. Combine the fruit in a blender.
4. Transfer the contents of the bowl to a serving glass and enjoy.

Easy Overnight Oats With Cinnamon

Ingredients:

- 1 1/2 tsp chia seeds

- 1 & 1/2 tsp pure maple syrup / brown sugar or as need

- 1/4 tsp cinnamon

- 1/4 tsp vanilla or almond flavoring

- 1/2 cup of + 2 tbsp almond milk

- 1/3 cup of old fashioned oats

- 1 cup of almond milk

- 3/4 cup of old fashioned oats

- 1 tbsp chia seeds

- 1 tbsp pure maple syrup

- 1/2 tsp cinnamon

- 1/2 tsp vanilla extract

Directions:
1. In a 12 ounce jar, mix all of the INGREDIENTS:.
2. Place the lid on the jar and shake it to stir the INGREDIENTS:. Make the oats are well mixed with almond milk.
3. Refrigerate for 8 hours.
4. Without the addition of fresh fruit, it will keep for 3-5 days. Fresh fruit, granola, almonds, or coconut can be added to the mix.

Pear, Ginger And Almond Yogurt Parfait

Ingredients:

- 1 tsp minced ginger
- 2 tsp honey
- ½ cup of sliced almonds
- 2 pears
- 3 cups of greek yogurt

Directions:

1. Pears should be peeled, cored, and diced into small chunks.
2. In a mixing bowl, add the pear and Greek yogurt, along with the ginger and, if desired, a drizzle of honey.
3. Serve with sliced almonds on top.

Energy Cookies With Oats And Raisins

Ingredients:

- The zest of a grated orange

- 150 g of rice malt

- A teaspoon of ground cinnamon

- A teaspoon of vanilla powder

- Apple juice to taste

- 300 g of rolled oats

- 100 g of raisins

- The grated zest of a lemon

Directions:

1. First, soak the raisins in warm water for about 15 minutes, turn on the oven at 180 ° and

prepare a pan lined with parchment paper to lay the biscuits to cook them.
2. Once this is done, you can dedicate yourself to the dough, starting with toasting the oat flakes in a hot pan for a few minutes, stirring often.
3. Place them still hot in a large bowl in which you will add the grated citrus peel, cinnamon, vanilla powder, and finally, the well squeezed raisins.
4. At this point, add the malt to the mixture; knead with your hands with the help of a little apple juice (just enough to be able to work the dough without making it too liquid).
5. You can proceed by taking some of the dough to form balls that you will crush in your hands to give it the classic shape of a round biscuit.
6. During this step, you can help yourself by wetting your hands with water.

7. Place each biscuit in the pan and bake for about 10-15 minutes.
8. Remove the pan from the oven and let the cookies cool.

9. When they are cold, you can store them in an airtight jar, where they will keep well for a whole week.

Soft Fruit Plumcake

Ingredients:

- 2 egg whites
- the zest of 1 grated lemon
- 1 jar of low-fat yogurt
- 100 g of shelled walnuts
- fresh berries (blueberries, currants, raspberries)
- 300 g of buckwheat flour
- 80 g of sugar
- 1 sachet of yeast
- 5 tablespoons of oil

Directions:

1. Mix the flour, sugar, oil, and yeast in a bowl, stir in the yogurt and lemon zest.
2. Separately, whisk the egg whites and add them gently to the previous INGREDIENTS:.
3. Finally, mix the walnuts and berries into the mixture.
4. Line a loaf pan with baking paper and pour the mixture.
5. Bake at 180 degrees for about 40 minutes.
6. If you want, you can serve this dessert with more low-fat yogurt and some fresh fruit.

Spiced Stuffed Peppers

Ingredients:

- 2 twigs new parsley, minced
- 1 teaspoon coriander seed, broke
- Tabasco sauce, to taste
- 1 teaspoon dried thyme
- Salt and ground dark pepper, to taste
- 1 cup cooked basmati rice
- 2 extra-enormous chime peppers
- 2 tablespoons olive oil
- 1/4 cup finely cleaved red onion
- 1 clove garlic, minced

- Nonstick cooking splash, depending on the situation

- 2 cups canned puréed tomatoes

- 2 tablespoons ground Parmesan cheese

Directions:

1. Heat olive oil on medium-low in a medium skillet.
2. Mix in onions and garlic, and sauté for 4 minutes.
3. Add parsley, coriander, Tabasco, thyme, salt, and pepper.
4. Whenever very much blended, spoon in rice, mixing to cover with oil, spices, and spices.
5. Preheat stove to 350°F. Daintily splash a shallow baking dish with cooking spray.
6. Cut each pepper in half the long way, and eliminate stems and seeds.
7. Load up with rice blend. Pour puréed tomatoes over the top.

8. Sprinkle with Parmesan cheese. Bake for 35 minutes.

Flank Steak With Chimichurri

Ingredients:

- ½ teaspoon sea salt, divided
- 1 (12-ounce) flank steak
- 3 tablespoons olive oil, divided
- ½ cup chopped fresh parsley
- ¼ cup chopped fresh cilantro
- 1 teaspoon dried oregano
- 1 teaspoon ground cumin
- Grated zest of ½ lime

Directions:
1. In a small bowl, stir together the oregano, cumin, and 1/4 teaspoon of salt.
2. Sprinkle evenly all over the flank steak.

3. Heat 1 tablespoon of oil in a large nonstick skillet over medium-high heat until it shimmers.
4. Add the flank steak and cook for 2 to 3 minutes per side.
5. Reduce the heat to low. Continue cooking until the steak it reaches 135°F for medium-rare, about 5 minutes more.
6. Meanwhile, in a blender or food processor, combine the remaining 2 tablespoons of oil, parsley, cilantro, lime zest, and remaining 1/4 teaspoon of sea salt. Pulse 20 times, or until it is well combined.
7. Slice the flank steak thinly slices against the grain. Serve with the chimichurri.

Low Fodmap Coleslaw

Ingredients:

- 2 spring onions, green part only
- A small handful of fresh mint
- Olive oil
- Lemon juice
- ¼ a cabbage
- 1 carrot
- 1 stalk of celery
- Salt & pepper

Directions:

1. Cut the cabbage into several smaller pieces.
2. Peel and top the carrot. Cut into smaller pieces.

3. Chop the celery into 8 pieces.
4. Chop up the green of the spring onions a little.
5. Place all the vegetables in a food processor and process into small pieces.
6. Tip them all out into a serving bowl.
7. Drizzle over olive oil and lemon juice.'Season to taste.
8. Mix well and serve.

Oatmeal-Crusted Rosemary Salmon

Ingredients:

- 1 Tbsp white miso paste
- 10 sprigs rosemary (stems removed, chopped fine)
- 5 Tbsp dry oatmeal
- 1 Tbsp canola oil
- 2 lbs salmon filet (trimmed, skinless, pin bones removed, cut into 8-oz portions)
- 1 tsp lemon zest

Directions:
1. In a small bowl, mix the lemon zest, miso paste, and rosemary.
2. Brush it over the salmon and let sit in the refrigerator, covered, for 5 minutes or up to 2 hours.

3. Remove the salmon from refrigerator.
4. Dip the presentation side (usually the side with the pin bones) into the oatmeal, which will adhere to the miso-lemon mix.
5. Heat a large non-stick pan over medium heat.
6. Add the oil and, when sizzling, add the salmon.
7. Lower the temperature slightly and cook until the oatmeal turns golden brown, approximately 5–7 minutes.
8. Flip with a wide non-stick spatula and cook another 5 minutes.
9. Drain on a paper towel to remove excess fat.
10. Serve over a salad or with a vegetable of your choice.

www.ingramcontent.com/pod-product-compliance
Lightning Source LLC
Chambersburg PA
CBHW071457080526
44587CB00014B/2130